T0311489

Cambridge Elements ≡

Elements of Improving Quality and Safety in Healthcare
edited by
Mary Dixon-Woods,* Katrina Brown,* Sonja Marjanovic,
† Tom Ling,† Ellen Perry,* Graham Martin,* Gemma Petley,* and
Claire Dipple*
*THIS Institute (The Healthcare Improvement Studies Institute)
†RAND Europe

DESIGN CREATIVITY

Gyuchan Thomas Jun,[1] Sue Hignett,[1] and
P. John Clarkson[2]
[1]*School of Design and Creative Arts, Loughborough University*
[2]*Engineering Design Centre, Department of Engineering, University of Cambridge*

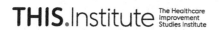
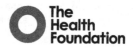

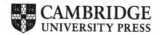

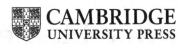

Shaftesbury Road, Cambridge CB2 8EA, United Kingdom

One Liberty Plaza, 20th Floor, New York, NY 10006, USA

477 Williamstown Road, Port Melbourne, VIC 3207, Australia

314–321, 3rd Floor, Plot 3, Splendor Forum, Jasola District Centre,
New Delhi – 110025, India

103 Penang Road, #05–06/07, Visioncrest Commercial, Singapore 238467

Cambridge University Press is part of Cambridge University Press & Assessment,
a department of the University of Cambridge.

We share the University's mission to contribute to society through the pursuit of
education, learning and research at the highest international levels of excellence.

www.cambridge.org
Information on this title: www.cambridge.org/9781009325332

DOI: 10.1017/9781009325318

First published 2024

A catalogue record for this publication is available from the British Library.

ISBN 978-1-009-32533-2 Paperback
ISSN 2754-2912 (online)
ISSN 2754-2904 (print)

Design Creativity

Elements of Improving Quality and Safety in Healthcare

DOI: 10.1017/9781009325318
First published online: May 2024

Gyuchan Thomas Jun,[1] Sue Hignett,[1] and P. John Clarkson[2]
[1]*School of Design and Creative Arts, Loughborough University*
[2]*Engineering Design Centre, Department of Engineering,*
University of Cambridge

Author for correspondence: P. John Clarkson, pjc10@cam.ac.uk

Abstract: Design creativity describes the process by which needs are explored and translated into requirements for change. This Element examines the role of design creativity within the context of healthcare improvement. It begins by outlining the characteristics of design thinking, and the key status of the Double Diamond model. It provides practical tools to support design creativity, including ethnographic/observational studies, personas, and scenarios, and needs identification and requirements analysis. It also covers brainstorming, Disney, and six thinking hats techniques, the nine windows technique, morphological charts and product architecting, and concept evaluation. The tools, covering all stages of the Double Diamond model, are supported by examples of their use in healthcare improvement. The Element concludes with a critique of design creativity and the evidence for its application in healthcare improvement. This title is also available as Open Access on Cambridge Core.

Keywords: creativity, design thinking, idea generation, personas, requirements analysis, healthcare, improvement, quality, safety, outcomes

ISBNs: 9781009325332 (PB), 9781009325318 (OC)
ISSNs: 2754-2912 (online), 2754-2904 (print)

Contents

1 Introduction

Improving healthcare requires good design at multiple levels and stages. In 2017, Royal Academy of Engineering's report, *Engineering Better Care – A Systems Approach to Health and Care Design and Continuous Improvement*,[1] highlighted design as one of four 'key perspectives' necessary for delivery of effective care (the others are people, systems, and risk). Design is especially important in answering three key questions:

- What are the needs?
- How can the needs be met?
- How well are the needs met?

Answering any or all of these questions may require creativity. In this Element, we focus on *design creativity*. Though it is sometimes mistakenly understood as the process for developing novel and useful ideas, solutions, or products,[2] design creativity can be defined more broadly to encompass the wider process of understanding the problem as well as solving it. With its origins in design thinking and design process, design creativity can be thought of as both the means to explore needs for improvement and the means to create new concepts in response to those needs. So, design creativity refers to the process of designing ('design' as a verb) rather than just the output of design ('design' as a noun).

Simon[3] has defined design broadly by saying that to design is to devise 'courses of action aimed at changing existing situations into preferred ones'. *Design science* is the study of the principles, practices, and procedures of design:[4,5] it aims to understand and improve how designers work and think, it establishes an appropriate structure for the design process, and it develops new design methods, techniques, and procedures for various design problems. These problems are often ill-defined, ill-structured, or 'wicked',[6] similar to many quality and safety issues in healthcare. Many design studies have looked at how the design process is managed to deliver consistently successful results and what methods and tools are applied.

We begin by outlining the characteristics of design thinking, the key status of the Double Diamond model, and the role of design creativity on healthcare improvement. We then review a range of tools that may be used to support design creativity.

In order to fully appreciate creativity as the process that enables teams to define the right problem and provide the best solution, this Element should be read alongside Elements on systems mapping[7] and risk assessment.[8]

1.1 Characteristics of Design Thinking

The history of design is almost as long as that of human history: people have either crafted objects (artefacts) or have found someone to do it for them. During the Industrial Revolution of the eighteenth and nineteenth centuries, rapid innovation led to the separation of design and making (manufacturing).[9] In contrast to the artisans of the past, post-Industrial Revolution designers had to meet the needs of large populations. They had to consider functionality, aesthetics, and usability, and balance the needs of manufacturers, including manufacturability, cost, and marketability. By the middle of the twentieth century, the need to combine engineering design and psychology had become more apparent – for example, in improving the design of aircraft controls and displays based on an understanding of human (e.g. pilot) and environmental factors.[10] This recognition led to the development of human factors/ergonomics as its own field of study and, in 1949, to the formation of the Ergonomics Society UK (now the Chartered Institute of Ergonomics and Human Factors). Human factors/ergonomics focus on designing the systems with which people interact in physical, organisational, and social environments in order to improve human well-being and system performance.[11]

Human factors and ergonomics were important in the development of user-centred design philosophy and processes. These processes aim to make the needs, wants, and limitations of the end user the priority focus, and offer a range of methods and techniques to ensure this focus is sustained through the various stages of design. Inclusive design, which emerged in the mid-1990s, encourages designers to create products and services that 'address the needs of the widest possible audience, irrespective of age or ability'.[12] It is defined as 'design of mainstream products and/or services that are accessible to, and usable by, people with the widest range of abilities within the widest range of situations without the need for special adaptation or design'.[13]

Designers rely on a distinctive way of thinking: design has its own way of problem-solving that is different from humanities and science.[4,14] Research into understanding design thinking began in the 1970s by looking at how designers form images in their minds and then manipulate and evaluate those ideas before, during, and after expressing them.[14] Design thinking has been described as applying a designer's sensibility and methods to problem-solving, no matter what the problem is.[15] Alluding to earlier work by Rittel and Webber on 'wicked' problems,[6] Cross has characterised design thinking in the following way: 'The designer's task is to produce 'the solution' in order to cope with ill-defined problems. The designer has to learn to have the self-confidence to define, redefine and change the problem-as-given in the light of the solution that emerges from their mind and hand'.

Developing creative ideas is one of the strengths of this way of thinking. Over the years, researchers have attempted to identify influences on creativity and how to support creativity in the design process. Some of the interesting questions explored by different design researchers have included: 'How do designers develop new ideas?', 'How do their ideas evolve?', and 'How do they move from one idea to the next?'.[16]

What design research has found so far is still very limited, but some findings are relevant to the development of improvement ideas in healthcare. When generating ideas, designers use their background experiences and skills, as well as different types of internal and external stimuli.[17] Internal stimuli are drawn from a person's working and long-term memories and may take the form of mental imagery or verbal information. External stimuli, on the other hand, are drawn from a person's surroundings and may include pictorial, verbal, audible, or tangible objects, for example.[18] External stimuli can be the result of actively seeking information (deliberately searching for particular information via the internet or in books, for example) or of a passive encounter (randomly encountering relevant information).

Research has also shown that exposing people to previous ideas can have a dual effect on new idea development:[19] it can be both positive, with inspirational sources stretching the potential pool of creative solutions,[19] and negative, limiting ideas to the replication of aspects of existing ideas and examples. This negative impact is called fixation.[16] Professional designers may try to prevent fixation by adopting some or all of the following approaches: promoting teamwork to avoid isolated individual work; use of systematic design methods; use of expert facilitation during idea-generation sessions (to control any negative effects of group behaviour); making and testing models and prototypes; and expecting concept variety.[20]

As designers and those not trained in design work increasingly alongside each other in co-design processes,[21] the importance of scaling up from individual to collective creativity is now recognised, with new definitions of design thinking emerging. For instance, Tim Brown, CEO of the global design and innovation company IDEO, has described design thinking as a human-centred approach to innovation that draws from the designer's toolkit to integrate the needs of people, the possibilities of technology, and the requirements for business success.[22] He also highlights that design thinking can be used by anyone to create breakthrough ideas.[22]

1.2 The Double Diamond Model

An especially important innovation in design thinking is the Double Diamond model (Figure 1),[23] which offers a framework for the design and delivery of

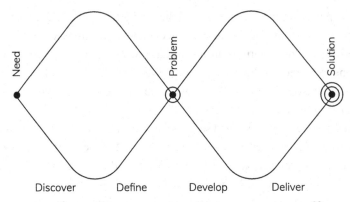

Figure 1 The Double Diamond design process model[23]

products, services, and systems. Developed by the UK Design Council in 2005, and describing a holistic process of creativity, it was originally derived from the observation of a wide range of real design processes. The research on which the Double Diamond is based focuses on those attributes of design thinking that had led to significant commercial success, rather than identifying and avoiding those that led to failure. It is widely cited as a model for capturing the essence of good design practice.

The Double Diamond design process model (Figure 1) identifies four core activities:

- Discover: explore current needs and solutions, and gather insights into the challenge.
- Define: balance the range of needs and articulate a clear statement of the challenge to be resolved.
- Develop: generate and evaluate solutions to the challenge.
- Deliver: launch the new organisation, product, or service.

The shape of the model has a particular meaning: it highlights the importance of translating need into a statement of challenge before developing solutions. It illustrates the value of exploration (or divergent thinking) before refinement (or convergent thinking). Each activity is a key element of the overall creative process, and each requires real creativity to deliver meaningful results. This underlines the importance of exploring the full range of stakeholder needs for improvement before balancing and refining those (often conflicting) needs into a clear statement of the challenge. It also emphasises the importance of exploring a wide range of possible concepts and potential solutions before committing to a particular solution and the means to deliver it into practice.

Improvement practitioners in healthcare may use a range of improvement methods and tools, including, as described throughout this Elements series, the Model for Improvement, Lean, Six Sigma, total quality management, business process reengineering, supply chain management, and many others. All of these methods require effective approaches to ensure effective problem-understanding and problem-solving. The importance of understanding the real needs for a system before delivering new solutions is illustrated by the challenges faced when introducing a new computerised command and control system for the London Ambulance Service (Box 1).

Despite the value of design thinking for improvement, it has been relatively slow to penetrate healthcare – apart from areas such as medical devices. This means that the design creativity required for optimising improvement approaches may not always be clearly stated. For instance, one of the three questions in the Model for Improvement is, 'What change can we make that will result in improvement?'. To answer this effectively, the needs for change (and their context) must be fully understood and change ideas that can lead to improvement must be generated. The Institute for Healthcare Improvement proposes that specific changes can be developed from a limited number of what it calls 'change concepts': general notions or approaches to change that have been found to be useful in developing more specific ideas for changes that can lead to improvement.[24] An example of a change concept is error proofing, which involves designing or re-designing systems to make it less

---

BOX 1 LONDON AMBULANCE SERVICE

Following an earlier failure in the 1980s, a comprehensive effort began in 1990 to define the requirements for a new and ambitious, state-of-the-art, and computerised command and control system for the London Ambulance Service.[1] The concept behind the design was that most calls would automatically be allocated to the most appropriate ambulance without the need for a human allocator. The new service was delivered in 1992 and immediately failed. Lessons learnt were that the particular geographical, social, and political environment in which the service operated, and the cultural climate within the service itself, required 'a more measured and participative approach' from management and staff. After several further attempts, a new system successfully went live in March 2012. While the fully automated allocation system met its operational expectations, contributory factors to earlier failures were thought to include poor understanding of paramedic behaviour, limited understanding of whole system performance, and inadequate preparation and risk assessment for system roll-out.[1]

likely for people in the system to make errors.[24] Other tools for developing change ideas widely used in healthcare include driver diagrams,[25] which offer a visual illustration of how specific change ideas or activities are connected with structures, processes, goals, and outcomes of the overall system. However, neither change concepts nor driver diagrams typically make enough use of creativity methods to fully understand the needs for change or to generate new change ideas that will result in improvement. In the next section, we describe tools that can be used to support design creativity in healthcare improvement.

2 Tools for Design Creativity

Design creativity plays a crucial role both in understanding an existing system and in the development of new systems. In the former, often referred to as re-design, the objective is to understand and enhance what already exists ('as is'). In the latter, often known as original design, the goal is to create what is intended to exist ('to be') and document the final outcome. The creative elements of design processes underlying both design and re-design have developed over many years, as have the tools that have emerged to support them. This section presents a selection of these tools, including:

- ethnographic/observational studies
- personas and scenarios
- needs identification and requirements analysis
- brainstorming, Disney, and six thinking hats
- the nine windows technique
- morphological charts and product architecting
- concept evaluation.

The tools described here are a small selection of the many available; they are chosen to provide a useful starting point for anyone with limited design experience and to cover all stages of the Double Diamond model.

2.1 Ethnographic Studies or Observational Studies

Ethnography is a research method for social sciences and anthropology which investigates customs, social behaviour, and human culture in specific settings. The methods of ethnography have been evolving to reflect the changing demands of health research,[26] but traditional ethnography in cultural anthropology requires the researcher to observe a culture for enough time (perhaps several months or years) to learn about the norms and values of the people in that setting.[27]

Design ethnography often starts with a series of observations in a specific setting before a new product, service, or system is developed. Observational methods can be casual (unstructured), semi-structured, or structured and systematic. Semi-structured and casual observations are typically used in the exploratory phase of the design process to collect baseline information through immersion; structured and systematic observations, on the other hand, typically use pre-structured worksheets, checklists, or codes to guide the observation. A variety of methods can be used to guide structured observations – for example, the AEIOU (Activities, Environments, Interactions, Objects, and Users) framework (Table 1) helps to structure observations by offering a classification system along with relevant questions as described in the table.[28] The AEIOU framework can be used in creative workshops with stakeholders to converge relevant information onto a large worksheet for data synthesis and design ideation.

Data for design ethnography are collected using qualitative research methods – interviews, observations, note-taking, video, and photography. They are analysed using a qualitative approach, such as open-ended discovery of patterns within discourse or by mapping data to categories of interest to the design inquiry.[29] A method like affinity diagramming (Figure 2) is often used to organise and structure data.[29]

Another method that can be used with structured observations is link analysis (Figure 3). This method aims to analyse physical interactions – human to human,

Table 1 Observation worksheet – AEIOU Framework

A – Activities
What are people doing?
E – Environment
What is the role of the environment?
How are people using the environment?
I – Interactions
Do you observe special interactions between people or between people and
    objects?
Do you see any routines?
O – Objects
What objects are there and are they being used or not used?
Are there any workarounds you can identify?
U – Users
Who are the users you are observing? What are their roles?
Are there any extreme users?

Adapted from Lewrick et al.[28]

Random ideas   Affinity diagram

Theme 1   Theme 2   Theme 3

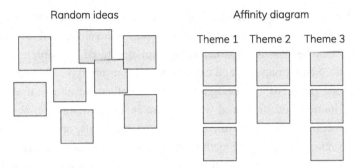

Figure 2 Affinity diagram for structuring/clustering random ideas

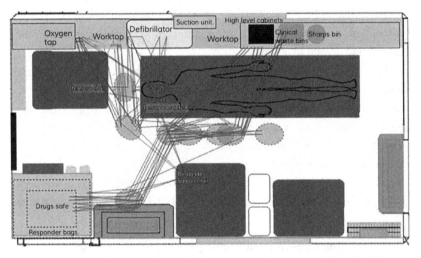

Figure 3 Link analysis showing movements of a paramedic technician
(bulkhead door layout)[34]

human to machine/environment, and machine to machine/environment – as
components within a system or product as structured observations. Link analysis
can be used to identify problems and to improve the layout of a working environment or a control panel, for example. It uses a data (event) recording method to
input interactions of human behaviour with their environment. A link occurs
when an individual shifts attention or physically moves from one part of the
system to another.[30] Link analysis enables understanding of how different parts of
the interface or system are linked to each other.[31] The case study in Box 2
describes how the method was applied in the development of a national specification for emergency ambulances within the UK National Health Service (NHS),
while Figure 3 illustrates the use of link analysis to show the movements of
a paramedic within an ambulance.

Box 2 Link analysis in developing a national specification for emergency ambulances

In 2003, a programme of human factors and ergonomics research began with the aim of standardising the design of emergency ambulances. The project was a response to the challenge that different NHS ambulance trusts were using individual vehicle specifications, resulting in over 40 different designs of emergency ambulances in the UK. This presented an increased risk to patient safety, as the interior layout and the location of equipment and consumables varied between vehicles, with the resulting impact on safe systems of work and efficiency of clinical care.

The research included observations and link analysis to compare ambulance loading systems[32] and an evaluation of vehicle and equipment risks for both paramedics and bariatric (obese) patients.[33] The findings provided an evidence base for a national specification for emergency ambulances, with nine areas of design recommendations: access/egress (exit), space and layout, securing people and equipment in transit, communication, security, violence and aggression, hygiene, vehicle engineering, and patient experience.[33] The national specification for emergency ambulances in 2006 was able to draw on this evidence base and incorporated 80 per cent of the recommendations.

The nine design criteria were used in 2023 by the London Ambulance Service NHS Trust with professional human factors specialists from Loughborough University to review the integration of new ambulance technologies (a powered stretcher and powered chair).

2.2 Personas and Scenarios

Personas are fictitious representations of target users[35] created from information collected from real users through field research such as ethnographic studies. Personas describe archetypal (rather than actual) people and their common behaviour patterns in meaningful and relatable profiles. As a technique, personas can provide useful design targets and facilitate empathy and communication during the ideation phase of the design process, when ideas and concepts are formed. Personas are typically presented in one or two pages, and feature a fictitious name for the person, a photograph, and a narrative that describes in detail key aspects of his or her life situation, goals, and behaviour relevant to the design inquiry.[28]

Personas can be used to support designers' ideation and co-designing in stakeholder workshops. For example, a persona called Jeff, a 77-year-old man, was created for co-design workshops with 30 stakeholders (clinicians, social care workers, pharmacists, and commissioners) that aimed to develop safer integrated medicine management systems.[36] Jeff was developed from interviews with 10 stakeholders (before the workshop) and presented at the workshop to help participants stand in the shoes of users and focus on resolving real user needs. Box 3 sets out some of the key information created about Jeff.

Another example is a set of five dementia personas developed and validated with clinicians, care providers, and designers (architects). The personas represent the symptoms, care needs, and design needs of people at different stages of dementia:[37] Alison (new diagnosis), Barry (thinking about moving into a care facility), Christine (living in a care facility), Chris and Sally (living at home), and David (end of life, living in a care facility).

These five personas were created through an iterative development and review process. Initial versions were created from a systematic literature review and scoping study ($n = 113$) to consider activities of daily living that might be relevant to or important for people with dementia (eating, toileting, social interaction, and physical activity), and to recommend design solutions to support these activities. This was followed by an iterative cycle of interviews, focus groups, and care environment observations with clinicians, care providers, and designers (architects) to create, review, and evaluate the personas. The final five personas were created in three formats: 2D matrix, 3D wheel, and five short films with actors playing the patients.

The five personas were used in the design process for adapting a two-up two-down Victorian terraced house to support independent living for people with different stages of dementia. By highlighting symptoms, care needs, and design needs (see Figures 4 and 5), the personas helped to create a shared mental model that the multidisciplinary team could use to consider design options and review decisions when assessing whether or not a design was likely to be suitable and

---

Box 3 Key details from the persona of Jeff

Jeff lives alone in North London on the second floor of a tower block that has no lift. Jeff quit smoking a few years ago but has reduced mobility (he uses a scooter), and he spends most of his time watching TV. Jeff has two grown-up children who live in Manchester and visit once or twice a year. His medical history includes chronic obstructive pulmonary disease, type 2 diabetes, hypertension, and mild depression. Jeff currently takes eight different medications at different times of the day. A local community pharmacy arranges repeat prescriptions for Jeff and delivers medications to his home each month.[36]

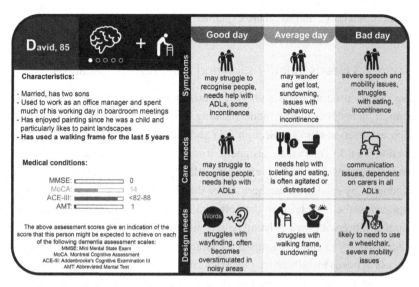

Figure 4 David persona: later stage of vascular dementia through to end of life[38]

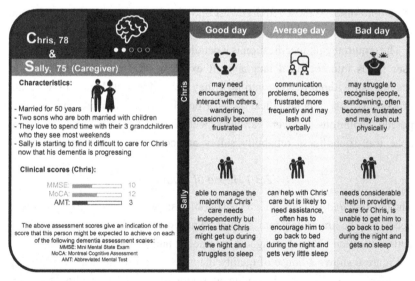

Figure 5 Chris and Sally (couple) personas for the dementia house[38]

whether future changes may be needed to maintain a supportive environment. The five personas supported the creation of an adaptable environment that is suitable for people at different stages of dementia and on good, average, and bad days.[37] Aspects of the design approach, layout, colour scheme, product, furniture selection, and so on are explained and illustrated in five short films of the personas with patient actors.[39]

2.3 Needs Identification and Requirements Analysis

The design process starts with the identification of users' needs. Designers commit themselves to truly understanding those needs by employing methods such as observations (see Section 2.1) and the creation of user personas (see Section 2.2). In contrast to designers, it is worth noting that many traditional innovation consultants often rely on so-called user interviews, which are often conducted by market researchers rather than the consultants themselves. This approach sometimes leads to the potential for selective information gathering, aligning more with their existing beliefs and expectations.[37] Designers, on the other hand, try to embody a mindset characterised by pure curiosity during the process of needs identification. Once this crucial phase of needs identification is firmly established, designers can go on to specify the objectives that the proposed solutions should fulfil, a step known as requirements analysis.

Tizani[40] has described design as a prolonged process of checking and pondering what may be often quite contradictory requirements, and making a series of compromises on those requirements until the design is achieved – as the end product of numerous associations of ideas ('a network of ideas').

The requirements specification is a detailed description and translation of the user needs into technical language. It explains what the solutions need to accomplish without delving into how they will achieve it. Later in the design process, we use this specification as a benchmark to measure and evaluate potential solutions. It covers various aspects, including functionality, performance, user-friendliness, reliability, safety, and compliance with regulations.

2.3.1 House of Quality

The *house of quality* diagram is a visual tool to show in a matrix format how user needs can be translated into system requirements. It provides a means of communication between designers, engineers, and various stakeholders.[41]

Figure 6 shows a house of quality diagram for a private healthcare setting where a survey had been conducted to measure service quality.[42] In this example, the lower part of the diagram highlights the relationships between patient needs ('Whats') and the functional requirements ('Hows') of the service, while the upper part (roof) shows the correlations between these functional requirements ('Hows'). It is apparent from the first row of the matrix (shaded in dark grey in Figure 6) that there is a strong relationship between the skills of doctors, the behaviour and attitude of staff, having modern equipment available,

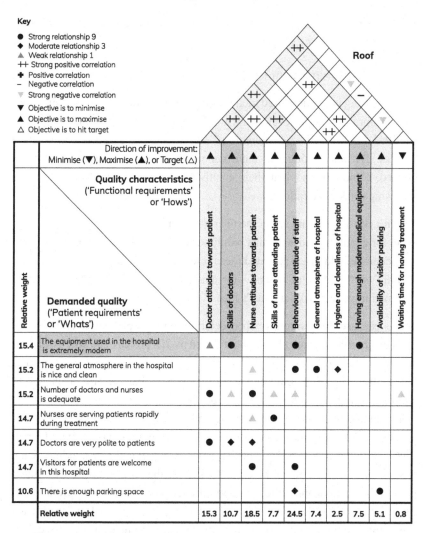

Figure 6 House of quality for a hospital

Adapted from Camgöz-Akdağ et al.[42]

and patients' requirement for modern equipment to be used. There is a weaker relationship between the attitudes of doctors and the use of modern equipment, which reflects that the modernisation of equipment has a slight effect on doctor attitude. The correlations between the technical requirements indicate, for example (as shaded in light grey in Figure 6), that doctor attitudes towards patients have a strong positive relationship with attitude and behaviour of nurses, attitude and behaviour of other staff, and availability of visitor parking. It might be argued that these relationships and correlations are obvious (which may be the case), but the fact that they are made explicit in the house of quality highlights their importance in understanding the problem and in developing requirements and ideas for improvement.

2.4 Brainstorming, Disney, and Six Thinking Hats

Brainstorming is a widely used method for generating ideas in a group situation. Alex Osborn originally developed it and first coined the term brainstorming. In his 1953 book, *Applied Imagination*,[43] he attempted to codify the creative process. By researching the environment in which his advertising teams worked, Osborn found that their creativity was most stimulated when the following rules were followed:

- Don't edit what's said and remember not to criticise ideas.
- Go for quantity of ideas at this point; narrow down the list later.
- Encourage wild or exaggerated ideas (creativity is the key).
- Build on the ideas of others – for example, one team member might say something that sparks another's idea.[43]

Teams can use brainstorming when determining possible causes and/or solutions to a problem, when planning out the steps of a project, and when deciding which problem (or opportunity) to work on. A brainstorming session typically has a 30-minute time limit but ends when everyone has had a chance to participate, and no more ideas are being offered.

Techniques to support brainstorming include the *Disney* method. Developed by Robert Dilts,[44] it was inspired by the innovative thinking that Walt Disney (1901–66) used in his strategic business development and film-making. When Disney had an idea for a film, he looked at the idea from at least three perspectives and adapted them as appropriate: producer (how to produce the film), director (how the film will come across on the screen), and audience (what aspects the audience will like or dislike). The method helps a team to look at problems from different perspectives and generate ideas accordingly. The Disney method uses the following three perspectives and roles for ideation:

- Dreamer: being creative and imaginative, seeing limitless opportunities
- Realist: looking at the practical possibilities to find out whether an idea is really feasible, considering the resources available
- Critic: looking at a plan, identifying any barriers and filtering out all crucial mistakes rather than criticising the initial dreams.

The perspectives and roles can be used at the same time or in sequence. For example, the brainstorming session can be run with an assumption that the roles of dreamer, realist, and critic will each be adopted in turn.

Six thinking hats is a variant of the Disney method. Created by Edward de Bono,[45] and based on the principle of parallel thinking, it aims to help those involved in the design process to adopt different ways of thinking by taking off their normal hat and wearing another. The process works best when a time limit (a maximum of 4 or 5 minutes) is imposed for wearing each hat. The six hats and relevant questions are as follows:

- White hat (data needs): what data do we have or need?
- Black hat (risk): what could go wrong?
- Yellow hat (benefits): what are the benefits?
- Green hat (ideas): how could the idea be developed further?
- Red hat (emotion): what do you feel about this?
- Blue hat (thinking process): what are the findings so far, and what needs to happen next?

2.5 Nine Windows Technique

The *nine windows* technique is an ideation tool for examining problems, exploring potential solutions, and identifying available resources in the dimensions of time and system. It does this by examining the past, present, and future at different system levels, including super-system level and related subsystems. The technique was developed by Genrich Altshuller,[46] creator of the TRIZ methodology (TRIZ is the Russian acronym for TIPS, Theory of Inventive Problem Solving).

Instead of only thinking about a problem and potential solution in terms of the present and at system level, the nine windows technique also prompts teams to explore a problem in the past and possible future and at both super-system and subsystem levels (see Figure 7). The team can zoom in to the product/service at the subsystem level or zoom out and consider the super-system. The team can consider changes from what happened in the past to what might happen in the future. This approach helps overcome barriers and see the product and service from a different point of view.[28]

2.6 Morphological Charts and Product Architecting

Creativity can take many forms – from an inspired idea for a whole product to the choice of material for a component within a complex system, or the novel teaming of people in the delivery of a new service. All have their place. But when product and service needs (and solutions) become more complicated, designers and design teams may need the support of a structured approach to concept generation. Not only will this help to widen the search for potential

	Past	Present	Future
Super-system	Paper-based patient folder	Electronic patient record	Access control by patient
System	Centralised database	Decentralised database	Distributed database
Subsystem	Paper, poster storage	Hospital computers	Any computers

Figure 7 Nine windows technique
Adapted from Lewrick.[28]

solutions, but it also provides a framework for informing the early stages of concept evaluation.

Morphological charts[47] are a visual way of representing possible design solutions by mapping design ideas against the core features or functions that a product or service is required to deliver. Designers are encouraged to identify as many alternative ideas as possible and then, by selecting combinations of those ideas, to form design concepts that are most likely to meet the requirements. This allows for exploration of alternative product architectures that may be appropriate in realising the product. The visual nature of morphological charts also encourages user involvement at an early stage of the design process when their influence can be most effective.

The process of building a morphological chart begins with identifying a moderate number (6–12) of key features or functions that a product must have but in a form that does not limit the nature of the design solution (so, for example, 'dose entry' rather than 'keypad'). These can be arranged in groups (providing some structure or architecture to the product) where they are likely to share common elements of a solution. Ideas are then sought to make each feature or function happen, taking care to list a range of possibilities rather than variations on a theme, and arranged in rows alongside the features and functions. Design concepts are then formed when viable combinations of ideas (one from each row) are selected.

The morphological chart in Figure 8 shows an example of the output of a brainstorming activity focused on the specific functional needs of face mask design. Any one of the approaches described previously could have been used to help generate this sort of idea.

Morphological charts have been applied to a wide range of domains over the years, from engineering design to policy analysis,[49] and they have a long history of application to healthcare planning, for example, in the design and evaluation of healthcare systems for a large metropolitan community.[50]

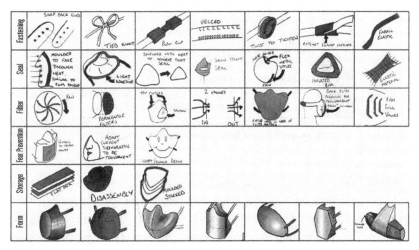

Figure 8 An example of a morphological chart for face mask design[48]

2.7 Concept Evaluation

Concept evaluation involves checking that a proposed concept (or concepts) not only meets the requirements of an improvement intervention but also meets the underlying needs of the patients or care providers. Concept evaluation can take different forms, reflecting the stage of the design process and the level of description of the concept at that point in time. But in all cases, its purpose is to judge the quality of the concept in terms of its match to the needs and requirements of the design solution.[51]

In broad terms, the purpose of evaluation may be thought of as testing the concept against defined requirements (often known as verification) or measuring its fitness for purpose in meeting real needs (known as validation).[51] For example, verification of an asthma inhaler tests its fit to documented device requirements, whereas validation measures its ability to deliver an appropriate dose of drug to the patient under typical conditions of use. Verification and validation may be summarised as respectively asking, 'Are we doing the thing right?' and 'Are we doing the right thing?'. Both are essential for product and service development and improvement, but verification is best suited to concept evaluation when it is assumed that some definition of requirements has already been completed.

Evaluation takes place at multiple levels. For example, there are things a new product or service must be able to do, and evaluation is needed to determine whether an individual concept is able to meet those demands and, therefore, whether it is viable. There may also be other things that may be desirable for a new product or service to do, and evaluation is then focused on the extent to which it is able to do so.

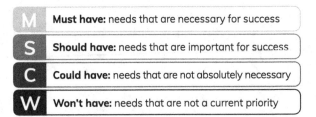

Figure 9 MoSCoW prioritisation of needs

Several tools are available to assist with concept evaluation. One is the MoSCoW prioritisation technique (Figure 9), which uses four categories – must have, should have, could have, and will not have[52] – as a means of comparing the relative merits of competing concepts. As before, the first of these provides a 'gate' or minimum standard for a concept, while the next two provide potential for comparing concepts and their ability to maximise delivery of the requirements. However, these comparisons aren't meant to provide a specific preferred formula for a concept. Instead, they point out the relative strengths and weaknesses between competing concepts. Evaluation methods have become more visible in health and care service design with the formation of the Health Product People[53] community in 2018 to bring together people working on digital services across the health and care space to share ideas, collaborate, and work together to solve problems. The community builds on the good work of the cross-government product and service community, which was formed to ensure that government products and services meet user needs. The blog referenced [53] presents a variety of narratives describing methods, such as human-centred design and design evaluation, and their relevance to improvement of digital health services.

3 Critiques of Design Creativity

The Royal Academy of Engineering, the Royal College of Physicians, and the Academy of Medical Sciences have all highlighted how design creativity can be showcased for those involved in healthcare improvement.[1] The advent of experience-based design approaches has also emphasised the role of users and stakeholders in co-understanding improvement challenges and co-designing solutions. However, formal evidence to demonstrate the effectiveness and cost-effectiveness of these approaches is lacking, since this is not an area known for its use of formal evaluation methods, such as randomised control trials to evidence success. Case studies, user feedback, and testimonials or expert opinions are often used to present the effectiveness of design creativity approaches, but providing concrete evidence is challenging. This is due to issues including the subjectivity and complexity of design outcomes, the diverse objectives of applying approaches, and the high level of context dependency of the findings. Instead, creativity in systems and product design has a long history of relevance in engineering design, which is typically evidenced by commercial success. As a result, literature of this form is scarce, with publications normally more narrative in form. The same is true for the application of creativity techniques in health and care improvement, and further research is needed to better evidence the value of creativity in improvement. However, design thinking has gained widespread acceptance and has been adopted by numerous organisations in various industries. It is important to note that the effectiveness of these design creativity approaches can vary depending on the context, project goals, and the skill of the team applying them.

Nonetheless, a systematic review of the impact of a systems approach to health and care improvement has been undertaken and suggests that a systems approach to healthcare design and delivery results in a statistically significant improvement to both patient and service outcomes.[54] In this context, a systems approach is defined as one that integrates perspectives on people, systems, design, and risk in a way that is applicable to healthcare systems across all scales from local service systems through to organisational, cross-organisational, and national policy levels. A further study found little evidence of understanding within the health service of the value and significance of design – especially in relation to managing and implementing design improvements to improve patient safety.[55] The authors found cause to question not simply the design of medical devices, products, packaging, and information but the way the health service as a whole uses, or rather fails to use, design in an effective way, and also fails to understand what design thinking can bring to an organisation.

There is much to be done to introduce creativity, in its broadest sense, to improvement practice, in particular by bringing a new perspective to enable more effective improvement. Some methods, such as observational studies, personas, and brainstorming, are already used to a limited extent in healthcare improvement, but a wider and more systematic application would likely be valuable. There is far less evidence of application within healthcare of some other methods, such as house of quality (see Section 2.3.1), morphological charts (Section 2.6), and MoSCoW prioritisation charts (Section 2.7), all of which will require the collaboration of experienced design practitioners.

3.1 Making Exploration Explicit

Improvement practices and design practices have each influenced the other, and both have adopted some methods that originated with the other. But healthcare can benefit even further by embracing the design thinking methods introduced in this

Element. Some research suggests that the 'explore' stage of the design process (i.e. exploring the ill-defined problem space before generating concept solutions – the first diamond in the Double Diamond model in Figure 1) should be conducted more explicitly in the healthcare improvement process.[56,57] Observation studies in combination with the AEIOU framework, affinity diagram and link analysis (see Section 2.1), and personas (see Section 2.2) can support this stage in particular. These methods can enable multiple stakeholders, including patients and healthcare providers, to explore potential issues and conflicts.

3.2 Idea Generation and Organisational Culture

The 'idea generation' stage in improvement uses change principles and process maps, but further use of a broad range of divergent thinking methods (the divergent part of the second diamond in the Double Diamond model – Figure 1), such as brainstorming, Disney, and six thinking hats (see Section 2.4), nine windows (see Section 2.5), and morphological charts (see Section 2.6), can help to generate a wider range of options.

However, such idea-generating methods only work in organisations that develop and nurture a culture of creativity and innovation. Considerable evidence shows that intrinsic motivation is more powerful in driving up levels of creativity than external motivators, such as competition, expected evaluation, or rewards.[58]

Nurturing a culture of idea generation (and possibly innovation) in a target-driven, performance-managed healthcare system is a major challenge,[59] not least because a top-down approach may undervalue stakeholder involvement and decrease intrinsic motivation. Divergent thinking can also be difficult to encourage in organisations that prioritise action and don't allow much time (or where little time is available) to explore a problem before implementing a solution, or where the challenge spans multiple departments or organisations. So, healthcare organisations should think carefully not only about how to exploit divergent thinking methods but also how to develop and nurture an innovative culture in the long term. Healthcare managers, while attending to policy changes, can also consider what they might do to support an innovative culture. Organisational support (e.g. time, resources, training, skills) and management support (e.g. attentiveness, coaching, giving useful feedback, being open to criticism) are all critical to the enhancement of innovative culture in healthcare.[60]

3.3 Evaluation

The 'evaluation' stage in design process (the convergent part of the second diamond in the Double Diamond model – Figure 1) involves assessing a wide range of ideas against goals and constraints to decide on the most appropriate final concept.

Small-scale and short-term piloting (i.e. new ideas are quickly tested, adjusted, and implemented into practice) is widely used in healthcare improvement. But while rapid piloting may be appropriate for some interventions, it is not the only approach to evaluation – and it can be problematic in some circumstances, particularly where there is uncertainty as to the risks that may be introduced by change.

Using MoSCoW prioritisation (see Section 2.7) to evaluate new ideas and concept solutions before piloting and implementation can help staff to identify and address issues before they emerge. Various physical, virtual, and conceptual evaluations can also be carried out in the design process before implementation – for example, types of system analysis, such as fault tree analysis, worst case analysis, what-if analysis, and failure mode and effect analysis (see the Element on risk assessment[8]). Computer-based scenario simulation approaches may also be useful in evaluating potentially high-risk concepts before they are implemented.[61,62]

3.4 Incorporating Design into Improvement

Introducing designers and design principles into the health and care environment has the potential to accelerate the adoption of creativity methods and tools. Many of the design methods and tools introduced in this Element are most likely to be most effective when multidisciplinary teams, including designers themselves, are involved in their application. An example of such practice is the Helix Centre[63] (a research lab for design and health co-founded by Imperial College London and the Royal College of Art) located at St Mary's Hospital in London, which describes itself as 'a studio space for designers, clinicians and patients to come together to explore and develop new ideas that positively impact healthcare delivery'. This immersion approach captures the essence of the Double Diamond model, where as much effort is spent in understanding the problem as finding the right solution. Other hospitals are turning to their clinical engineering teams to provide a similar design service, for example, the Clinical Engineering Innovation team and Cambridge University Hospitals[64] that aim to identify novel, unmet clinical needs and translate these into innovative medical technologies and processes to benefit patients, staff, and the wider health economy. Whilst much narrative evidence exists on the value of design-led approaches in improvement, further research is required to directly link improved or altered outcomes to design creativity interventions.

4 Conclusions

Creativity is needed for exploring needs for improvement, creating novel and workable solutions for improvement, and evaluating their success. Activities and tools developed and applied by design researchers and practitioners have the potential to add considerable value in improving healthcare. When appropriately used, the design methods and tools introduced in this Element can support development of human-centred, innovative, and sustainable solutions.

Design creativity is more than a way of thinking: it's also a set of structured principles and approaches. The Double Diamond model presented in this Element is an example of a framework that emphasises the importance of exploration, creativity, and evaluation in contributing to the successful delivery of change or improvement. A toolkit of design methods, a sample of which has been shown here, then facilitates the delivery of creativity within the improvement process. This way of thinking is relevant to all improvement and is intended to complement and supplement existing methods and approaches to improvement.

5 Further Reading

Buckle et al.[65] – outlines a view of the NHS from a fresh standpoint, applying the design approach and experience of other safety-critical industries to deliver a clear message: that the NHS needs to think in broad design and system terms much more so than it does at present.

Brown and Martin[66] – explains the beginning of design thinking to improve the process of designing tangible products. The Intercorp story presented in this review shows that design thinking principles have the potential to be even more powerful when applied to managing the intangible challenges involved in getting people to engage with and adopt innovative new ideas and experiences.

Burns et al.[67] – introduces RED, a 'do tank' that challenges accepted thinking. It designs new public services, systems, and products that address social and economic problems. These problems are increasingly complex and traditional public services are ill-equipped to address them. Innovation is required to reconnect public services to people and the everyday problems that they face.

Clarkson et al.[1] – this report, co-produced with engineers, clinicians, and healthcare leaders, explores how an engineering approach could be applied in health and social care to develop systems that meet the needs of patients, carers, and NHS staff. It presents a new framework to support ongoing work in service design and improvement in health and care.

Cottam and Leadbeater[68] – a guide to the Design Council–established RED, a new unit challenging accepted thinking on economic and social issues through design innovation. It ran rapid live projects to develop new thinking and practical design solutions in the form of systems, services, and products.

Design Council[69] – an in-depth study of the design processes used in 11 global brands. The results give an insight into the way design operates in these firms and delivers usable lessons for all designers and managers.

Kolko[70] – covers principles that include a focus on users' experiences, especially their emotional ones; the creation of physical models, such as diagrams and sketches, to explore problems; the use of prototypes to experiment with solutions; a tolerance for failure; and thoughtful restraint in product features so that even a complex piece of technology can be easy to use.

Contributors

All authors contributed significantly to the development of this Element. All authors have approved the final version.

Conflicts of Interest

None.

Acknowledgements

We thank the peer reviewers for their insightful comments and recommendations to improve the Element. A list of peer reviewers is published at www.cambridge.org/IQ/peer-reviewers.

Funding

This Element was funded by THIS Institute (The Healthcare Improvement Studies Institute, www.thisinstitute.cam.ac.uk). THIS Institute is strengthening the evidence base for improving the quality and safety of healthcare. THIS Institute is supported by a grant to the University of Cambridge from the Health Foundation – an independent charity committed to bringing about better health and healthcare for people in the UK.

About the Authors

Gyuchan Thomas Jun is a professor of socio-technical system design at the School of Design and Creative Arts, Loughborough University, and a chartered ergonomist and human factors specialist. His research interest has been in applying systems thinking approaches to the design of complex healthcare systems and integrating new technologies into healthcare systems.

Sue Hignett is a professor of healthcare ergonomics and patient safety at the School of Design and Creative Arts, Loughborough University. She is a Fellow of the Chartered Institute of Ergonomics and Human Factors and a chartered physiotherapist. Her research looks at a wide range of human factors and ergonomics issues.

P. John Clarkson is the Director of the Cambridge Engineering Design Centre and Co-Director of Cambridge Public Health. His research interests are in the general area of engineering design, particularly the development of design methodologies to address specific design issues, for example, process management, change management, healthcare design, and inclusive design.

Creative Commons License

References

1. Clarkson J, Bogle D, Dean J et al. *Engineering Better Care – A Systems Approach to Health and Care Design and Continuous Improvement.* London: Royal Academy of Engineering; 2017. https://raeng.org.uk/media/wwko2fs4/final-report-engineering-better-care-version-for-web site.pdf (accessed 20 December 2023).
2. Sarkar P, Chakrabarti A. Assessing design creativity. *Des Stud* 2011; 32(4): 348–83. http://dx.doi.org/10.1016/j.destud.2011.01.002.
3. Simon HA. The science of design: Creating the artificial. *Sci Artif* 2020; 4(1/2): 67–82. https://doi.org/10.2307/1511391.
4. Cross N. The nature and nurture of design ability. *Des Stud* 1990; 11(3): 127–40. https://doi.org/10.1016/0142-694X(90)90002-T.
5. Cross N. Designerly ways of knowing: Design discipline versus design science. *Des Issues* 2001; 17(3): 49–55. www.jstor.org/stable/1511801.
6. Rittel HWJ, Webber MM. Dilemmas in a general theory of planning. *Policy Sci* 1973; 4(2): 155–69. https://doi.org/10.1007/BF01405730.
7. Komashie A, Kotiadis K, Lamé G, Clarkson P. Systems mapping. In Dixon-Woods M, Brown K, Marjanovic S et al., eds. *Elements of Improving Quality and Safety in Healthcare.* Cambridge: Cambridge University Press; forthcoming.
8. Card A, Ward J, Clarkson P. Risk assessment. In Dixon-Woods M, Brown K, Marjanovic S et al., eds. *Elements of Improving Quality and Safety in Healthcare.* Cambridge: Cambridge University Press; forthcoming.
9. King S, Chang K. *Understanding Industrial Design.* Farnham: O'Reilly Media, Inc; 2018.
10. Waterson P, Eason K. '1966 and all that': Trends and developments in UK ergonomics during the 1960s. *Ergonomics.* 2009; 52(11): 1323–41. https://doi.org/10.1080/00140130903229561.
11. Hignett S, Carayon P, Buckle P, Catchpole K. State of science: Human factors and ergonomics in healthcare. *Ergonomics* 2013; 56(10): 1491–503. http://dx.doi.org/10.1080/00140139.2013.822932.
12. Clarkson J, Coleman R. History of inclusive design in the UK. *Appl Ergon* 2015; 46(Part B): 235–47. https://doi.org/10.1016/j.apergo.2013.03.002.
13. Institute BS. British Standard 7000–6:2005. Design Management Systems – Managing Inclusive Design – Guide. London: BSI; 2005. https://doi.org/10.3403/03208286U.

14. Archer B. Design as a discipline: Whatever became of design methodology? *Des Stud* 1979; 1(1): 17–20. https://doi.org/10.1016/0142-694X(79)90023-1.

15. Lockwood T. *Design Thinking: Integrating Innovation, Customer Experience and Brand Value.* New York: Allworth Press; 2009.

16. Crilly N. Creativity and fixation in the real world: A literature review of case study research. *Des Stud* 2019; 64: 154–68. https://doi.org/10.1016/j.destud.2019.07.002.

17. Gonçalves M, Cardoso C, Badke-Schaub P. What inspires designers? Preferences on inspirational approaches during idea generation. *Des Stud* 2014; 35(1): 29–53. https://doi.org/10.1016/j.destud.2013.09.001.

18. Eastman C. New directions in design cognition: Studies of representation and recall. In Eastman C, Newstetter W, McCracken M, eds. *Design Knowing and Learning: Cognition in Design Education.* Atlanta: Elsevier Science; 2001: 147–98. https://doi.org/10.1016/B978-008043868-9/50008-5.

19. Cai H, Do EYL, Zimring CM. Extended linkography and distance graph in design evaluation: An empirical study of the dual effects of inspiration sources in creative design. *Des Stud.* 2010; 31(2): 146–68. https://doi.org/10.1016/j.destud.2009.12.003.

20. Crilly N. Fixation and creativity in concept development: The attitudes and practices of expert designers. *Des Stud.* 2015; 38: 54–91. https://doi.org/10.1016/j.destud.2015.01.002.

21. Sanders EBN, Stappers PJ. Co-creation and the new landscapes of design. *CoDesign.* 2008; 4(1): 5–18. https://doi.org/10.1080/15710880701875068.

22. Brown T. Design thinking. *Harv Bus Rev* 2008; 86(6): 84–92. https://hbr.org/2008/06/design-thinking.

23. Design Council. Eleven lessons: Managing design in eleven global brands; 2005. www.designcouncil.org.uk/fileadmin/uploads/dc/Documents/ElevenLessons_Design_Council%2520%25282%2529.pdf (accessed 20 December 2023).

24. Langley GL, Moen R, Nolan KM et al. *The Improvement Guide: A Practical Approach to Enhancing Organizational Performance.* Oxford: John Wiley & Sons; 2009.

25. Institute for Healthcare Improvement. Quality Improvement Essentials Toolkit; 2017. www.ihi.org/resources/Pages/Tools/Quality-Improvement-Essentials-Toolkit.aspx (accessed 20 December 2023).

26. Waring J, Jones L. Maintaining the link between methodology and method in ethnographic health research. *BMJ Qual Saf* 2016; 25(7): 556–67. http://dx.doi.org/10.1136/bmjqs-2016-005325.

27. Hammersley M. Ethnography: Problems and prospects. *Ethnogr Educ* 2006; 1(1): 3–14. https://doi.org/10.1080/17457820500512697.

28. Lewrick M, Link P, Leifer L. *The Design Thinking Playbook: Mindful Digital Transformation of Teams, Products, Services, Businesses and Ecosystems*. Oxford: Wiley; 2018.

29. Martin B, Hanington BM. *Universal Methods of Design: 100 Ways to Research Complex Problems, Develop Innovative Ideas, and Design Effective Solutions*. Beverly, MA: Rockport Publishers; 2012.

30. Kirwan B, Ainsworth LK. *A Guide to Task Analysis*. Oxford: Taylor & Francis; 1992.

31. Shepherd A. *Hierarchical Task Analysis*. Oxford: Taylor & Francis; 2001.

32. Jones A, Hignett S. Safe access/egress system for emergency ambulances. *Emerg Med J* 2007; 24(3): 200–5. http://dx.doi.org/10.1136/emj.2006 .041707.

33. Hignet S, Griffiths P. Manual handling risks in the bariatric (obese) patient pathway in acute sector, community and ambulance care and treatment. *Work* 2009; 33(2): 175–80. http://dx.doi.org/10.3233/WOR-2009-0864.

34. Thorne, E. Development of a Protocol to Evaluate Ambulance Patient Compartments Using Link Analysis and Simulation. Unpublished BSc. dissertation. Dept of Human Sciences, Loughborough University; 2008.

35. Pruitt J, Adlin T. *The Essential Persona Lifecycle: Your Guide to Building and Using Personas*. London: Morgan Kauffman; 2006.

36. Jun GT, Canham A, Altuna-palacios A, Ward JR, Bhamra R. A participatory systems approach to design for safer integrated medicine management. *Ergonomics* 2018; 61(1): 48–68. https://doi.org/10.1080/00140139.2017 .1329939.

37. Jais C, Hignett S, Halsall W et al. Chris and Sally's house: Adapting a home for people living with dementia (innovative practice). *Dementia* 2021; 20(2): 770–78. https://doi.org/10.1177/1471301219887040.

38. Jais C, Hignett S, Galindo Estupiñan Z, Hogervorst E. Evidence based dementia personas: Human factors design for people living with dementia. In Polak-Sopinska A and Królikowski J, editors. *Ergonomics for People with Disabilities*. Poland: De Gruyter; 2018: 215–26. https://doi.org/ 10.2478/9783110617832-018.

39. Videos created to help families identify care needs of loved ones with dementia. www.lboro.ac.uk/news-events/news/2018/may/video-to-help-identify-demenetia-care-needs/ (Accessed 24 May 2023).

40. Tizani W. Engineering design. In Aouad G, Lee A, Wu S, editors. *Constructing the Future: nD Modelling*. Dordrecht: Routledge; 2006: 14–39. https://doi.org/10.4324/9780203967461.

41. Hauser JR, Clausing D. The house of quality. *Harv Bus Rev* 1988; https://hbr.org/1988/05/the-house-of-quality.

42. Camgöz-Akdağ H, Tarım M, Lonial S, Yatkın A. QFD application using SERVQUAL for private hospitals: A case study. *Leadersh Heal Serv* 2013; 26(3): 175–83. https://doi.org/10.1108/LHS-02-2013-0007.

43. Osborn A. *Applied Imagination.* New York: Charles Scribner's Sons; 1953.

44. Dilts R. *Strategies of Genius.* Capitola, California: Meta; 1994.

45. De Bono E. *Six Thinking Hats.* London: Penguin; 2000.

46. Altshuller G. *And Suddenly the Inventor Appeared: TRIZ, the Theory of Inventive Problem Solving.* Worcester, MA: Technical Innovation Center; 1996.

47. Zwincky F. The morphological approach to discovery, invention, research and construction. In Zwicky F, Wilson AG, editors. New Methods of Thought and Procedure – Contributions to the Symposium on Methodologies. Heidelberg: Springer Berlin; 1967; 273–97. https://doi.org/10.1007/978-3-642-87617-2.

48. Carter M, Lyle R, Watt K, Hogg J, Melville D. FFP3 facemask redesign. Industrial Group Project (DM403) Undertaken at the Department of Design, Manufacturing and Engineering Management, University of Strathclyde, in Partnership with Health Protection Scotland and NHS Health Scotland; 2016. https://issuu.com/matthewddcarter/docs/group_6_industrial_project_folio (accessed 15 January 2024).

49. Álvarez A, Ritchey T. Applications of general morphological analysis – From engineering design to policy analysis. *Acta Morphol Gen* 2015; 4(1): 1–40. www.swemorph.com/amg/pdf/amg-4-1-2015.pdf.

50. Turley RE, Richardson WC, Hansen JV. Morphological analysis for health care systems planning. *Socioecon Plann Sci* 1975; 9(2): 83–88. https://doi.org/10.1016/0038-0121(75)90013-0.

51. FDA. Design Control Guidance for Medical Device Manufacturers; 1998. www.fda.gov/media/116573/download (accessed 19 December 2023).

52. Clegg D, Barker R. Case Method Fast-Track: A RAD Approach. Boston: Addison-Wesley Longman; 1994.

53. Health Product People: Designing and Delivering Better Health and Care Digital Services. https://digitalhealth.blog.gov.uk/2018/11/12/health-product-people-designing-and-delivering-better-health-and-care-digital-services/ (accessed 1 February 2022).

54. Komashie A, Ward J, Bashford T et al. Systems approach to health service design, delivery and improvement: A systematic review and meta-analysis. *BMJ Open* 2021; 11(1): e037667. https://doi.org/10.1136/bmjopen-2020-037667.

55. Clarkson PJ, Buckle P, Coleman R et al. Design for patient safety: A review of the effectiveness of design in the UK health service. *J Eng Des* 2004; 15(2): 123–40. https://doi.org/10.1080/09544820310001617711.

56. Hignett S, Jones EL, Miller D et al. Human factors and ergonomics and quality improvement science: Integrating approaches for safety in healthcare. *BMJ Qual Saf* 2015; 24(4): 250–54. http://dx.doi.org/10.1136/bmjqs-2014-003623.

57. Jun GT, Morrison C, Clarkson PJ. Articulating current service development practices: A qualitative analysis of eleven mental health projects. *BMC Health Serv Res* 2014; 14. https://doi.org/10.1186/1472-6963-14-20.

58. Amabile TM, Schatzel EA, Moneta GB, Kramer SJ. Leader behaviors and the work environment for creativity: Perceived leader support. *Leadersh Q* 2004; 15(1): 5–32. https://doi.org/10.1016/j.leaqua.2003.12.003.

59. Massey C, Munt D. Preparing to be creative in the NHS: Making it personal. *Heal Care Anal* 2009; 17(4): 296–308. https://doi.org/10.1007/s10728-009-0132-1.

60. Cramm JM, Strating MMH, Bal R, Nieboer AP. A large-scale longitudinal study indicating the importance of perceived effectiveness, organizational and management support for innovative culture. *Soc Sci Med* 2013; 83: 119–24. https://doi.org/10.1016/j.socscimed.2013.01.017.

61. Jun GT, Morris Z, Eldabi T et al. Development of modelling method selection tool for health services management: From problem structuring methods to modelling and simulation methods. *BMC Health Serv Res* 2011; 11(108). https://doi.org/10.1186/1472-6963-11-108.

62. Ibrahim Shire M, Jun GT, Moon S, Robinson S. A system dynamics approach to workload management of hospital pharmacy staff: Modelling the trade-off between dispensing backlog and dispensing errors. *IISE Trans Occup Ergon Hum Factors* 2019; 6(3–4): 209–24. https://doi.org/10.1080/24725838.2018.1555563.

63. Helix Center. https://helixcentre.com/ (accessed 14 September 2023).

64. Clinical Engineering Innovation. www.cuh.nhs.uk/our-research/research-facilities/clinical-engineering (accessed 4 January 2024).

65. Buckle P, Clarkson PJ, Coleman R et al. *Design for Patient Safety: A System-Wide Design-Led Approach to Tackling Patient Safety in the NHS*, Department of Health and the Design Council, London; 2003.

66. Brown T, Martin R. Design for action: How to use design thinking to make great things actually happen. *Harv Bus Rev* 2015; 56–64. https://hbr.org/2015/09/design-for-action.

67. Burns C, Cottam H, Vanstone C, Winhall J. *RED Paper 02: Transformation Design*. Design Council, London; 2006.

68. Cottam H, Leadbeater C. *RED Paper 01 Health: Cocreating Services.* Design Council, London; 2004.

69. Design Council. *Eleven Lessons Managing Design in Eleven Global Companies.* Design Council, London; 2007.

70. Kolko J. Design thinking comes of age. *Harv Bus Rev* 2015; 66–71. https://hbr.org/2015/09/design-thinking-comes-of-age.

Cambridge Elements ☰

Improving Quality and Safety in Healthcare

Editors-in-Chief

Mary Dixon-Woods

THIS Institute (The Healthcare Improvement Studies Institute)

Mary is Director of THIS Institute and is the Health Foundation Professor of Healthcare Improvement Studies in the Department of Public Health and Primary Care at the University of Cambridge. Mary leads a programme of research focused on healthcare improvement, healthcare ethics, and methodological innovation in studying healthcare.

Graham Martin

THIS Institute (The Healthcare Improvement Studies Institute)

Graham is Director of Research at THIS Institute, leading applied research programmes and contributing to the institute's strategy and development. His research interests are in the organisation and delivery of healthcare, and particularly the role of professionals, managers, and patients and the public in efforts at organisational change.

Executive Editor

Katrina Brown

THIS Institute (The Healthcare Improvement Studies Institute)

Katrina was Communications Manager at THIS Institute, providing editorial expertise to maximise the impact of THIS Institute's research findings. She managed the project to produce the series until 2023.

Editorial Team

Sonja Marjanovic

RAND Europe

Sonja is Director of RAND Europe's healthcare innovation, industry, and policy research. Her work provides decision-makers with evidence and insights to support innovation and improvement in healthcare systems, and to support the translation of innovation into societal benefits for healthcare services and population health.

Tom Ling

RAND Europe

Tom is Head of Evaluation at RAND Europe and President of the European Evaluation Society, leading evaluations and applied research focused on the key challenges facing health services. His current health portfolio includes evaluations of the innovation landscape, quality improvement, communities of practice, patient flow, and service transformation.

Ellen Perry

THIS Institute (The Healthcare Improvement Studies Institute)

Ellen supported the production of the series during 2020–21.

Gemma Petley

THIS Institute (The Healthcare Improvement Studies Institute)

Gemma is Senior Communications and Editorial Manager at THIS Institute, responsible for overseeing the production and maximising the impact of the series.

Claire Dipple

THIS Institute (The Healthcare Improvement Studies Institute)

Claire is Editorial Project Manager at THIS Institute, responsible for editing and project managing the series.

About the Series

The past decade has seen enormous growth in both activity and research on improvement in healthcare. This series offers a comprehensive and authoritative set of overviews of the different improvement approaches available, exploring the thinking behind them, examining evidence for each approach, and identifying areas of debate.

Cambridge Elements ⸗

Improving Quality and Safety in Healthcare

Elements in the Series

Collaboration-Based Approaches
Graham Martin and Mary Dixon-Woods

Co-Producing and Co-Designing
Glenn Robert, Louise Locock, Oli Williams, Jocelyn Cornwell, Sara Donetto, and Joanna Goodrich

Implementation Science
Paul Wilson and Roman Kislov

Making Culture Change Happen
Russell Mannion

Operational Research Approaches
Martin Utley, Sonya Crowe, and Christina Pagel

Simulation as an Improvement Technique
Victoria Brazil, Eve Purdy, and Komal Bajaj

Workplace Conditions
Jill Maben, Jane Ball, and Amy C. Edmondson

Governance and Leadership
Naomi J. Fulop and Angus I. G. Ramsay

Health Economics
Andrew Street and Nils Gutacker

Approaches to Spread, Scale-Up, and Sustainability
Chrysanthi Papoutsi, Trisha Greenhalgh, and Sonja Marjanovic

Statistical Process Control
Mohammed Amin Mohammed

Values and Ethics
Alan Cribb, Vikki Entwistle, and Polly Mitchell

Design Creativity
Gyuchan Thomas Jun, Sue Hignett, and P. John Clarkson

A full series listing is available at: www.cambridge.org/IQ

Printed in the United States
by Baker & Taylor Publisher Services